The 14-Day Rapid Fat Loss Diet

A simple 2-week plan proven to target belly fat, melt inches, and produce rapid lasting results in your body and health!

By: Dr. Kristen Harvey

Congratulations on investing in the 14-day Diet!

As a thank you, I'd love to give you a BONUS 7 days on the Rapid Fat Loss Diet for FREE to help you get even better fat-melting, body-tightening results:

"The Un-edited 21-Day Rapid Fat Loss Diet Schedule"

You can download it right here: http://bit.ly/14daybook

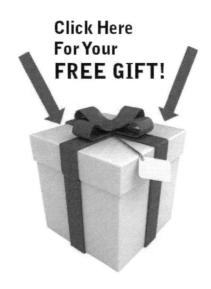

ABOUT THE AUTHOR:

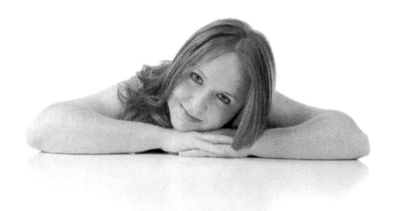

Dr. Kristen Harvey's passion for fitness started at a very early age, but it wasn't until she transformed her body, losing over 60 lbs., that she knew it would become her life's mission.

And for the last several years, Dr. Harvey and her husband have been helping transform the lives and bodies of 100's of clients through their fitness business, Scenic City Boot Camp and Transformation Center.

With over 20 years combined experience in the fitness industry, the Harvey's are passionate about finding new, exciting ways to make food and fitness fun so that everyone will CRAVE a healthy lifestyle.

The Harvey's have appeared on ABC, CBS, NBC, and Fox, consulted for companies such as Sherwin Williams, the University of TN, and the TN Dept of Education and are co-authors of the best-selling book, "The Wellness Code". They were also voted #1 in Personal Training in 2011 and 2013.

Dr. Harvey graduated as a Doctor of Physical Therapy in 2007 and holds several certifications in personal training, sports nutrition, healthy cooking, and functional movement.

Her 2020 vision is to help elevate and empower 1,000,000 overweight women to take back control of their life and transform their bodies from the inside out, using the same "effortless transformation" principles she used to dramatically change her body and life.

Why You Should Read This Book:

It might not seem clear to you right now but the 14-day diet is the most essential diet tool that you might ever stumble across to help you get control of your body and health FAST!

Why? Because it delivers POWERFUL results in just 14 days.

As a personal trainer and fitness expert, I've tried everything and seen everything... but nothing delivered my clients dramatic results like the 14-day diet. I've used it to help my clients drop from a size 12 to a size 6, lose up to 20 lbs., get into bikini-body shape, and win fitness contests, all while undergoing dramatic visible transformations (that they can literally see in the mirror!) in a matter of days.

The 14-day Rapid Fat Loss Diet is proven to target stubborn belly fat and produce lasting results. Most people report losing up to 3 inches off their bellybutton in 14 days and up to 6% body fat in 21 days (3x faster than the normal rate of fat loss!).

But the BEST news is- it's extremely simple to follow. You don't need a lot of time. You don't have to do much prep or cooking your meals ahead, and it's super easy to understand.

And while the 14-day diet is a rapid fat loss tool, its framework will help you understand how to eat for the rest of your life.

That's why I believe the 14-day diet is the ONLY diet you'll ever need.

So if you're frustrated and looking for a simple solution that will help you lose weight once and for all, then look no further, because you've finally found it!

Let's get started...

Disclaimer & Copyright Information

The contents are based on the author's personal experience and research. Your results may vary, and will be based on your individual situation and motivation.

There are no guarantees concerning the level of success you may experience. Each individual's success depends on his or her background, dedication, desire, and motivation.

I make every effort to ensure that I accurately represent our products and services. There is no guarantee that your results will match examples published in this report.

Some diet strategies may not work for many reasons beyond the control of the author. The author cannot guarantee or otherwise be responsible for your results using this plan.

Table of Contents

INTRODUCTION

Back in college, I was overweight, out-of-shape and just plain miserable. My eating had gotten out of control so I enlisted the help of a fitness coach. But she wasn't just ANY coach. She had dropped 60 lbs, after the birth of her 2 sons, and quickly became one of the most famous fitness models in the world.

Her weight loss success story inspired Oprah, E! and several other national media. That's when I heard about her. I knew that if I wanted to create results like she had done, the fastest way to do that was hire her as my coach. Little did I know, that decision would be one of the most life-changing and most important decisions of my life. Because not only did I completely transform my body, but that one decision changed the course of my career and my life. And today, the legacy is carried on as I share with you one of my most prized possessions from my weight loss journey; the 14-day Rapid Fat Loss Diet. My fitness coach gave me this 14-day plan to help me get into bikini body shape and I was blown away at how simple and effective it was. Since then, I've used this little "diet gem" to help hundreds of my boot camp and personal training clients unlock their stubborn fat stores and achieve dramatic results in a few short days. It's helped them get into bikini body shape, win body transformation contests, and get off blood pressure medications.

It's the same diet my fitness coach used to win the title of Miss Bikini America. And it's the same diet that I used to get into a 2 piece bikini for the first time in my life. And I believe this same diet will help you, too! Whether you're looking to kick-start your weight loss journey or lose the last 5 lbs., you'll find the 14-day diet to become one of your most valued tools in your weight loss "bag of tricks".

I hope you understand just how much POWER you hold in your hands, as this 14-day diet has changed hundreds of lives, and now it's YOUR TURN.

So... let's get started!

CHAPTER 1: JUST GIVE ME 14 DAYS...

Congrats! I'm so excited you've found this book. In the next few pages, I'm gonna share with you one of the most powerful diet strategies I've ever come across.

As a personal trainer, my career and reputation hinge on helping clients get results fast and in less time than anyone else.

The 14-day Rapid Fat Loss plan has become my tool of choice.

And today, it's your turn to put the 14-day Rapid Fat Loss diet to work for you.

So if you're ready to see dramatic changes in your body and burn body fat up to 3x faster than your average diet and fitness plan, then:

Give me your BEST effort for 14 days and you will get the BEST results you've ever gotten on a diet plan, PERIOD!

I know you're eager to get started, so let's begin!!!

CHAPTER 2: GETTING READY FOR THE 14-DAYS

#1- Know What You Want. #2- Know what is Important #3-Prioritize According to What is Important

Set your 14-day goal. With all challenges, no matter how big or small, it's important to have 2 things: 1) unwavering FOCUS that will allow you to exert all your energy on the task at hand, even when life gets in the way, and 2) an exciting and very specific goal of what you want to accomplish. Why is this important? Goals are the equivalent to putting blinders on a horse. The only thing they see is the path ahead of them and they stay laser-focused on the road ahead to get to the destination. So just like a horse with blinders, goals are your "vehicle" to move yourself to where you want to be. Obstacles are what you see when you take your eyes off your goals.

Now when setting your 14-day goal, make the goal emotionally-charged. Once you attach your emotions to the goal, your subconscious mind will start to work FOR you. So instead of a "# goal" like I'll drop 10 lbs., pull out your skinny jeans that you can't quite fit into right now (but you're close! Remember... this is only 14 days!) and use those to track your progress during the next 14 days. They'll probably hold a lot more significance to you than some abstract number on a scale that doesn't truly mean something to you.

WHAT IS REALISTIC TO ACHIEVE IN 14 DAYS?

On a typical weight loss plan, you can expect to lose 0.5-1% of body fat and 2-4 lbs. of fat in 2 weeks.

But this program is NOT your average plan. The 14-day plan is designed for those who don't want "ordinary" weight loss results. Why lose 1-2 lbs. per week when you can drop 10 lbs. in a week?

In order to get "uncommon results" you have to be willing to do "uncommon things", and so we will be tweaking things that you typically wouldn't do in a normal fat loss program. Nothing too extreme or drastic, but definitely challenging for some. Remember it's only 14-days, and as my training client told me, although it's not always "fun" to be on the diet, it is pretty awesome to see the scale drop everyday and notice changes in the mirror on a consistent basis.

Based on my clients who have done the 14-day or full 21-day plan, I have seen the following results:

Client #1: Size 12 to size 6 in 21 days.

Client #2: Lost 12 lbs. of pure body fat in 21 days.

Client #3: Unable to exercise due to medical problems but lost 12 lbs. in 10 days without exercise.

Client #4: Down 4 inches in the belly button and 2 inches in the hips.

Client #5: Lost 30 lbs. in 21 days.

Client #6: Lost 6% body fat in 21 days.

Client #7: Lost 3 inches off the hips and 3 inches off the waist in 14 days.

(While most people see the greatest results in the first 14 days, you can access the full 21-day schedule here for FREE: bit.ly/14daybook)

When setting goals, stretch your comfort zone but do not make them so unrealistic that your brain is telling yourself it is impossible.

Choose a goal that excites you and challenges you but is achievable (we are working in a very short time frame!).

Having an unusually large goal is an adrenaline infusion that provides the endurance to overcome the inevitable trials and tribulations that go along with any goal.

Because you will always get what you HAVE to have.

Put Your Goal in Stone. Get some 3x5 cards and keep one on your bathroom mirror, one on your night stand, one in your journal and one in your purse or your car. Remember, goals are your blinders. Your 14-day emotionally-charged goal is what will keep you going during this 14-day process even when you don't feel like it. Obstacles (other appointments, dinner with friends, etc.) are the things that throw you off track, when, and only when, you take your eyes off your goal.

You can do this! I believe you can do this! I know you can do this! It is only 2 weeks, or 14 days. It is YOUR choice whether you will eat the dinner rolls or choose the fish. It is YOUR choice whether you will cook your meals for the rest of the week on Sunday or hope to catch a good lunch on Monday.

CREATING A SUCCESSFUL MIND SHIFT:

There are 3 phrases that are NOT allowed during this 14 day period and hopefully not allowed back in your vocabulary long after this...

The words are "I can't", "I have to..." and "I'll try".

Instead, as soon as you say or think these words, replace them IMMEDIATELY with the words "I can.", "I GET TO" and "I'll do it!"

If you've failed on a diet in the past, remember, the past does not equal the future. It just means that the WAY it was approached may not have been the best strategy for success. So if we want to go after something we've never achieved before, we must be willing to do things differently than we have in the past.

RECORDING YOUR 14-DAY TRANSFORMATION:

Take a before picture. (Front/side/back)

Put on a bathing suit (trunks, 2-piece, 1-piece, or a sports bra and shorts.) Find a blank wall and make sure you are in a well-lighted area. Take a full-length shot (head to toe). Make sure it's clear!

Try to get your body fat tested before you start (scale at home with body fat or at your gym)

Take measurements. Bellybutton, hips, and chest are the most important ones.

Record your food in My Fitness Pal or another nutrition app. What gets measured gets managed. So if you want to see what you're eating to produce the results you're getting, make sure you write it down.

And like I mentioned earlier, find an article of clothing that is important to you (jeans, bikini, a certain t-shirt or dress) and use this to track your progress.

Your Nutrition TO-DO List

You will need to raid your pantry of "junk" and designate your kitchen as your "safe zone"

You will need to re-stock your kitchen with the foods on the meal plan on Sunday or Saturday

Follow the grocery list and the meal plan so that you can do your shopping and make sure you are ready. If there are things that you dislike on the plan, you will be given "substitutes" that you can choose to eat instead.

You will need to set aside some time on Sunday and possibly the middle of the week to plan, cook and prepare your meals so that they are easy to grab and eat during the day. Preparation is KEY in your success during the 14 days!

You will need to try to eat every 2-4 hours to keep your metabolism ROARING and to avoid any cravings. I guarantee you that a happy and satisfied tummy throughout the day will help control your cravings and help you ON A MAJOR LEVEL to make smart choices. If you go too long without a meal or snack, your blood sugar will drop, which often caters to ravenous cravings and grabbing the closest sugary snack or drink.

Small smartly-portioned meals eaten frequently throughout the day are like adding fuel to your metabolism, keeping it in HIGH GEAR, leading to a MAJOR calorie burn. Going without eating for a prolonged time period will SLOW your metabolism and sabotage your results.

Chapter 3: EASY TIPS TO BURN MORE FAT

Whenever you try to burn fat rapidly, you're going to need to do some "uncommon" things to get "uncommon but AMAZING results". So while we won't be covering the meal plan just yet, I do want to make sure you understand some of the basic principles behind rapid fat loss. Many of the tips below (including supplementation) are merely suggestions to help you maximize your results and aren't necessary for the 14-day diet, but if your budget allows, you may find some of these advanced tips and tools to further accelerate your results, as many of my clients did.

ADVANCED NUTRITION TIPS to ENHANCE your Fat-Burning Potential:

Dark leafy green vegetables and lean protein sources are a staple. Fish is one of the leanest sources of protein and yields the best fat loss results.

Healthy fats are essential on a high-protein, low-carb diet to keep your body healthy.

Drinking PLENTY OF WATER. You need to shoot for 1 gallon of water per day.

We'll be cutting out most wheat products, if not all.

For the 14 days, we'll try to stay away from dairy and alcohol. Alcohol is one of the biggest sabotagers of fat loss.

What you eat before bed is much more important than what you eat in the am. Do not eat starchy carbs (breads, pastas, etc.) within 6 hours of going to sleep. Better yet, make that 8 hours.

Do not go out to eat more than 1x per week.

If you're not already, start counting calories and macronutrients. While most fat loss plans recommend lower protein intake, for the purposes of rapid fat loss, a great goal is to shoot for approximately 0.8- 1.0 gram of protein per lb. of lean body weight.

Cleanse and Detox on the plan. My personal choice is Advocare's 10 day Metabolic Cleanse (To purchase, visit this website: http://www.advocare.com/10031858). In my opinion, it is easy, doesn't cause drastic changes in bathroom behaviors, and helps to detox the livers and kidneys, which helps the liver become more efficient at metabolizing fat. More importantly, during this diet, it is important to stay hydrated and the fiber drinks that come in the cleanse will help to slow down absorption rates of your food and water. It is $37 and highly recommended.

Now, a cheaper method is to drink a cleansing beverage 6-12 times per day (or add it to your water gallon) consisting of 8 oz. of water, 2 Tbsp. of fresh lemon juice (fresh squeezed, not refrigerated) and a pinch of cayenne pepper (which acts like little fans inside the blood to speed up metabolism). My favorite cleansing drink is the Flat Belly Diet's Sassy water, which you can find on my Pinterest Page under 14-day Recipes: www.pinterest.com/iconiclyfit.

"Fat Loss Stack" Supplementation:

Protein Powder. You will need a good protein powder. My personal preference is the Advocare Muscle Gain protein, found at the same website as the 10-Day Cleanse, because it is of superior quality, and pre-digested, meaning it is easy on your liver and kidneys, and easily absorbed. The MOST important thing to look for is something with less than 5-6 grams of carbs and less than 1 g of sugar. The Nectar brand is also one of my favorite brands of choice.

Multivitamin: If you are doing the 10-day cleanse, you will wait until the 10 days is over before you do a multivitamin. On a restricted diet plan, you want to make sure you are getting MAXIMUM nutrition via minimum calories. A good multivitamin is good for any plan, to fill in the gaps of your nutrition and make sure you are getting the nutrition you need.

Fish oil or Omega-3 supplements. They help to burn body fat (most notably, belly fat) support lean tissue, reduce inflammation, and support metabolism.

Catalyst: Commonly referred to as chicken breast in a bottle... Amino acids are the building blocks of protein and are a great supplement to take prior to a workout to support the maintenance of lean muscle tissue and fat burning. While this supplement is fantastic to include, don't get overwhelmed in the details. You must have whey protein for this plan. Your 2nd priority should be a multi-vitamin. Fish oil is extremely beneficial to have if you have the money. Catalyst should be the last on your list.

I know, from working with clients who are desperate for FAST results that they often want all the tools that they can get their hands on to maximize their results. So I'm spilling all the secrets in this section on how to maximize your fat-burning results, with additional tips and tools, but the 14-day diet in and of itself is AMAZING, so if you cannot afford to get supplements, don't worry! You're still going to hit it out of the park in terms of your weight loss results.

CHAPTER 4: The 14-day Diet in a Nutshell *(It's as easy as A, B, C)*

How the 14-day Diet Works...

You will cycle complex carbohydrates (sweet potatoes, brown rice, etc.) for 14 days following the guidelines and schedule below. This will allow your body to unlock your fat stores so you can launch a full-out attack for 14 days. The more made-from-scratch meals with simple ingredients and the less on-the-go items you choose, the better your results.

Day 1 is Plan A. Plan A is a 1-carb day meaning that you can only have complex carbs at breakfast. The rest of the day is lean proteins, fibrous carbs (vegetables) and whey protein shakes. All plans are described below the schedule with approved food lists and additional instructions below that.

14-Day Rapid Fat Loss Schedule:

- DAY 1   PLAN A
- DAY 2   PLAN A
- DAY 3   PLAN A
- DAY 4   PLAN B
- DAY 5   PLAN B
- DAY 6   PLAN C
- DAY 7   PLAN C
- DAY 8   PLAN B
- DAY 9   PLAN B
- DAY 10   PLAN B
- DAY 11   PLAN B
- DAY 12   PLAN A
- DAY 13   PLAN A
- DAY 14   PLAN C

Food Plan A- 1 Carb Day

Meal One
1 Protein
1 Complex Carb
1 Fibrous/Vegetable Carb

Meal Two
Shake

Meal Three
1 Protein
1 Fibrous/Vegetable Carb

Meal Four
Shake

Meal Five
1 Protein
1 Fibrous/Vegetable Carb

Meal Six
Shake

Food Plan B- No Carb Day

Meal One
1 Protein
1 Fibrous/Vegetable Carb

Meal Two
Shake

Meal Three
1 Protein
1 Fibrous/Vegetable Carb

Meal Four
Shake

Meal Five
1 Protein
1 Fibrous/Vegetable Carb

Meal Six
Shake

Food Plan C- 2 Carb Day

Meal One
1 Protein
1 Complex Carb
1 Fibrous/Vegetable Carb

Meal Two
Shake

Meal Three
1 Protein
1 Complex Carb
1 Fibrous/Vegetable Carb

Meal Four
Shake

Meal Five
1 Protein
1 Fibrous/Vegetable Carb

Meal Six
Shake

14-Day Guidelines

Build Your Plate Around Protein: You must have one at each meal! Recommended Serving Size: Approx. 4 oz. for women and 6 oz. for men.

Best sources of protein on the 14-day Diet are: Chicken breast, Turkey (extra-lean ground turkey breast, turkey bacon, turkey sausage, and turkey breast), fish and seafood, buffalo and wild game, extra-lean ground beef, and eggs.

My Recommendation: The leanest cuts of protein are the best. Fish trumps all lean protein sources, followed by chicken breast, eggs, and turkey breast. You will need a good source of whey protein powder (any flavor) with less than 5 g. of sugar and little to no sugar. You will need a protein shake (mixed with water) 3x a day!!!

Eat complex carbs at the recommended times on Plan A and Plan C days (NO COMPLEX CARBS on Plan B Days)

Sweet Potato trumps all other "complex carbs". You can never get fat off of sweet potato! You may get full or "spill over" but never fat! If you have to choose between eating brown rice and sweet potato, go for sweet potato!

A food scale is ideal to use.

Recommended Portions:
- *Sweet Potato* ~ ¾ cup
- *Brown Rice* ~½ cup

You can integrate other complex carbs into your diet such as squash and quinoa if you'd like but try to follow the guidelines as closely as possible. Absolutely no cereal or bread, unless it is Ezekiel bread.

Eat your veggies at every meal!

No: Corn, Carrots, Beets, or Peas!

Yes: Green leafy vegetables, broccoli, cucumber, asparagus, celery, green beans, onions, mushrooms, tomato and bell peppers.

CHAPTER 5: THE 14-DAY DONE-FOR-YOU MEAL PLAN

Please Note: The following is a suggested Meal Plan. You can stay "simple" and create your own meal plan, based on the above schedule (see 14-day schedule for details), or follow the suggested meal plan below.

14-DAY SUGGESTED MEAL PLAN

DAY 1 (1 carb)

Meal 1: 2 of Kristen's Grab 'n Go Egg Muffins, ½ c. brown rice

Meal 2: Protein Shake (mix with water)

Meal 3: 4-6 oz. grilled chicken (marinated in 10 min. Mrs. Dash) and salad (baby spinach (1 handful) mixed with mixed baby greens (1 handful), 1 tsp. olive oil, 1 tsp. red wine vinegar or balsamic vinegar

Meal 4: Protein Shake (mix with water)

Meal 5: Orange Roughy fish fillet, seared in frying pan with grapeseed oil, then seasoned to taste with broccoli (steamed)

Meal 6: Protein Shake (mix with water)

Day 2 (1 carb)

Meal 1: Southwest Veggie Omelet, ¾ c. baked sweet potato

Meal 2: Protein Shake

Meal 3: Lean Cuisine Steak Tips with Portobello & broccoli

Meal 4: Protein Shake

Meal 5: 4-6 oz. Maple-Soy salmon fillet, grilled asparagus with pinch of sea salt and pepper

Meal 6: Protein Shake

Day 3 (1 carb)

Meal 1: 1 slice Ezekiel bread with 1 Tbsp. extra-virgin coconut oil, 4-6 egg whites, 1-2 yolks, 1 strip turkey bacon, bell peppers, onions and mushrooms, chopped

Meal 2: Protein Shake

Meal 3: 4-6 oz. Maple-Soy salmon filet, grilled asparagus with pinch of sea salt and pepper

Meal 4: Protein Shake

Meal 5: Chicken Bruschetta with green beans

Meal 6: Protein Shake

Day 4 (0 carb)

Meal 1: 4-6 egg whites, 2 yolks, 1-2 strips turkey bacon, spinach, onions and mushrooms, chopped (1 slice of provolone cheese, if needed)

Meal 2: Protein Shake

Meal 3: 1 packet of Hickory-Smoked Tuna Creations, Green Salad with Avocados and 1 tsp. of lemon juice, 1 tsp of olive oil.

Meal 4: Protein Shake

Meal 5: Orange Roughy fish fillet, seared in frying pan with grape seed oil, then seasoned to taste with broccoli (steamed)

Meal 6: Protein Shake

Day 5 (0 carb)

Meal 1: Southwest Egg Scramble

Meal 2: Protein Shake

Meal 3: Grilled Chicken & Veggie Kabobs

Meal 4: Protein Shake

Meal 5: Jennie-O Turkey burgers or 5 oz. of extra-lean turkey breast, cooked as a burger in a fry pan, 1 cups Broccoli, 2 tsp Toasted Sesame Seed Oil, 2 TBSP Lite Soy Sauce

Meal 6: Protein Shake

Day 6 (2 carb)

Meal 1: ¾ c. Sweet potato fries, 4-6 egg whites, 2 yolks, 1-2 strips turkey bacon, bell peppers, onions and mushrooms, chopped

Meal 2: Protein Shake

Meal 3: Salmon Bowl: Captain Gorton Grilled Salmon fillet, ½ cup of 90 sec. Uncle Bens brown rice and 1 cup of spinach (frozen), all mixed together.

Meal 4: Protein Shake

Meal 5: Chicken Marsala with Braised Broccoli

Meal 6: Protein Shake

Day 7 (2 carb)

Meal 1: 1 slice Ezekiel bread with 1 Tbsp. extra-virgin coconut oil, 4-6 egg whites, 1-2 yolks, 1 strip turkey bacon, bell peppers, onions and mushrooms, chopped

Meal 2: Protein Shake

Meal 3: Lemon-Herbed Tilapia with Green Beans Provencal and ½ cup steamed brown rice

Meal 4: Protein Shake

Meal 5: Grilled Chicken Kabobs

Meal 6: Protein Shake

Day 8 (0 carb)

Meal 1: 4-6 egg whites, 2 yolks, 1-2 strips turkey bacon, bell peppers, onions and mushrooms, chopped

Meal 2: Protein Shake

Meal 3: Lean Cuisine Turkey and Green Beans

Meal 4: Protein Shake

Meal 5: Chicken Marsala with Braised Broccoli
Meal 6: Protein Shake

Day 9 (0 carb)

Meal 1: 2 Kristen's Grab 'n Go Egg Muffins

Meal 2: Protein Shake

Meal 3: Grilled Chicken Kabobs

Meal 4: Protein Shake

Meal 5: Balsamic Flank Steak with Sauteed Spinach and Faux Mashed Potatoes

Meal 6: Protein Shake

Day 10 (0 carb)

Meal 1: 4-6 egg whites, 2 yolks, 1-2 strips turkey bacon, bell peppers, onions and mushrooms, chopped

Meal 2: Protein Shake

Meal 3: Jennie-O Turkey Burger and Steam Fresh Brussel Sprouts

Meal 4: Protein Shake

Meal 5: Chicken Bruschetta with green beans

Meal 6: Protein Shake

Day 11 (0 carb)

Meal 1: 2 Kristen's Grab 'n Go Egg Muffins

Meal 2: Protein Shake

Meal 3: 4-6 oz. Maple-Soy salmon fillet, grilled asparagus

Meal 4: Protein Shake

Meal 5: Jennie-O Turkey Burger with Brussel Sprouts

Meal 6: Protein Shake

Day 12 (1 carb)

Meal 1: Southwest Egg Scramble, ¾ c. baked sweet potato

Meal 2: Protein Shake

Meal 3: Lean Cuisine Turkey and Green Beans

Meal 4: Protein Shake

Meal 5: 4-6 oz. Maple-Soy salmon fillet, grilled asparagus

Meal 6: Protein Shake

Day 13 (1 carb)

Meal 1: 1 slice Ezekiel bread, 3-5 egg whites, 1-2 yolks,2 slices turkey bacon, Bibb lettuce

Meal 2: Protein Shake (mix with water)

Meal 3: 4-6 oz. grilled chicken (marinated in 10 min. Mrs. Dash) and salad (baby spinach (1 handful) mixed with mixed baby greens (1 handful), 1 tsp. olive oil, 1 tsp. balsamic vinegar

Meal 4: Protein Shake (mix with water)

Meal 5: Orange Roughy fish fillet, seared in frying pan with grapeseed oil, broccoli (steamed)

Meal 6: Protein Shake (mix with water)

Day 14 (2 carb)

Meal 1: ¾ cup baked sweet potato, 3-5 egg whites, 1-2 yolks, 1-2 strips turkey bacon, bell peppers, onions and mushrooms, chopped

Meal 2: Protein Shake

Meal 3: Salmon Bowl: Captain Gorton Grilled Salmon fillet, ½ cup of Uncle Bens brown rice and 1 cup of spinach (frozen), all mixed together.

Meal 4: Protein Shake

Meal 5: Jennie-O Turkey Burger and Salad with 1 tsp. olive oil and 1 tsp. flavored vinegar of choice (or lemon juice)

Meal 6: Protein Shake

14-Day Recipes

Balsamic Flank Steak with Sautéed Spinach

& Faux Mashed Potatoes

- o   4-6 oz. Flank Steak
- o   2 Tbsp. Balsamic Vinegar
- o   2 Tsp. Olive Oil
- o   2 Tsp. Dried Rosemary, Minced
- o   1 cup spinach leaves, washed
- o   2 cups cauliflower florets, steamed until soft
- o   Nonstick cooking spray

Instructions: In a zip-top bag, combine the vinegar, oil and rosemary; add the flank steak into the bag and marinate for 30 to 60 minutes. Then cook steak on grill or in a broiler for about 4 minutes on each side. Meanwhile, heat a nonstick skillet coated with nonstick cooking spray over medium heat, and add spinach leaves; season with salt and pepper and sauté for 3 to 5 minutes. Lastly, blend the steamed cauliflower florets in a blender or food processor until smooth and then heat in the microwave.

Chicken Bruschetta

- 5 oz. boneless, skinless chicken breast, butter flied
- 1 tsp. onion powder
- 1 tsp. chili powder
- 1 plum tomato, diced
- 2 Tbsp. fresh basil, thinly sliced
- 1 tsp garlic, minced
- 1 tsp. olive oil
- 2 cups steamed green beans
- Salt and pepper to taste

Instructions: Season chicken with onion powder and chili powder, and grill or broil until done, about 4 to 5 minutes per side. To make bruschetta, combine tomatoes, basil and minced garlic and season with salt and pepper to taste. Top chicken with the bruschetta and serve with steamed green beans.

Chicken Marsala with Braised Broccoli

- 5 oz. boneless, skinless chicken breast, butter flied
- 1 tsp. Mrs. Dash Italian seasoning
- 2 Tbsp. chopped onion
- ½ cup sliced mushrooms
- 3 Tbsp. Marsala Wine
- 1 tsp. olive oil
- 1 tsp. dried rosemary
- 1 cup broccoli florets

Instructions: Butterfly your chicken breast by cutting it in ½ lengthwise. Season butterflied chicken breast with Mrs. Dash Italian seasoning. Heat a nonstick skillet sprayed with nonstick cooking spray over medium heat. Sauté chicken breast until cooked through and golden brown on each side- about 3 to 4 minutes per side. Remove chicken from pan and add olive oil, onion, mushrooms, and rosemary; sauté on medium-low heat for 3 to 4 minutes, until mushrooms begin to give off fluid. Add the marsala wine and simmer for 2 to 3 minutes, until reduced by half. Top chicken with marsala wine sauce. Meanwhile, steam the broccoli in the microwave for about 3 to 4 minutes, or until desired degree of softness.

Kristen's GRAB 'N GO Egg Muffins

- o 2 1/2 cups egg whites
- o 3 eggs
- o 6 slices of turkey bacon or 4-6 pcs of chicken or turkey sausage
- o 2 tablespoons of unsweetened almond milk (not necessary, but gives them a bit of fluff)
- o salt and pepper

Instructions

Preheat oven to 350 degrees F. Spray 12-cup muffin tin with nonstick cooking spray, you can also line with muffin tins, just make sure you spray the inside of the muffin tins.

1. Fill each muffin tin 1/4-1/3 full with veggies and herbs of choice. Add some turkey bacon or sausage to each muffin tin.

2. In medium bowl whisk together egg whites, eggs, and milk/yogurt. Fill each muffin to the top with egg mixture, pouring over the veggies already in each tin. Bake for 20-30 minutes or until risen and slightly golden on top.

3. Let cool for a few minutes

4. Remove from tin.

5. Put in Ziploc bag in refrigerator for grab and go meals every morning.

Lemon-Herbed Tilapia with Green Beans Provencal

- 6 oz. tilapia filet
- Juice of 1 lemon
- ½ tsp. dried thyme
- ½ tsp. dried rosemary
- 3 tbsp. brown rice bread crumbs
- 1 tsp. olive oil
- 1 cup green beans, steamed
- 4 Tbsp. marinara tomato sauce
- Salt and pepper to taste

Instructions: Preheat oven to 400 degrees. Spray an ovenproof dish with nonstick cooking spray and place tilapia filet in dish. Season the fish with salt and pepper. Then drizzle fish with olive and lemon, sprinkle with herbs, and dust with brown rice bread crumbs. Bake in the oven for 20 minutes or until fish flakes easily with a fork. Meanwhile, microwave the green beans and tomato sauce for 1 minute or until heated thoroughly.

Maple-Soy Grilled Salmon

- 1 Tbsp. Low-Sodium Soy Sauce
- 1 Tbsp. Pure Maple Syrup

Mix together soy sauce and maple syrup. Marinate salmon filet overnight. Grill until filet is tender enough that it breaks apart when touched with a fork.

Southwest Egg Scramble

- o 4-5 egg whites with 1 yolk
- o ¼ cup salsa
- o 1 strip of lean turkey bacon (or a Morningstar Stripple)
- o Green Bell Pepper, chopped
- o Onion, chopped
- o Mushrooms, chopped

Instructions: Heat up fry pan while mixing all the ingredients in a bowl. Cook like an omelette until done.

CHAPTER 6: THE 14-DAY DIET ON THE ROAD

Yes, even on the go, it is possible to stick to the 14-day diet. Although some sacrifices might be made, the 14 day rapid fat loss plan is pretty easy to follow while traveling, at business meetings, and when going out to eat.

When going out to eat, choose grilled chicken, salmon, and other grilled fish entrees with veggies or salad. Dressing and sauces should all be asked to be on the side.

Depending on where you are, do your homework before you go: go to www.calorieking.com and see how much calories your grilled chicken salad really does have at your favorite restaurant. Many restaurants offer online menus which you can look up before you go.

Planning ahead is key to your success!!!!

However, the bulk of your meals should be made at your hotel room. For best results, use the following convenience food list and most importantly, use the Semi-Homemade How-To to create the "best" on-the-go meals for BEST RESULTS.

ON THE ROAD AGAIN... Traveling by Car

What you need: A cooler.

What to do before you go: Pre-package fresh veggies, Pack bottles of water and a funnel so you can easily mix your protein shakes, divvy up your protein powder in little baggies (or use a funnel locker or Blender Bottle, found at GNC) for easy shake-it-up snacks, put salads and dressing in containers, pack easy lean protein options, pack your supplements and make sure to keep them in a cool, dry place.

ON THE ROAD AGAIN... In the Hotel Room

Always plan ahead and check to see if there is a refrigerator and microwave in your room. If not, ask if there is a way to get one in your room during your stay. In most cases, they should oblige. Make sure you pack some silverware and a Shaker cup for your protein shakes, or a small Magic Bullet blender (available at Target, Walgreens, Bed Bath and Beyond) to mix your protein shakes quickly and easily.

You might also want to bring a container to bring meals with you as well for when you are away at meetings or busy.

Spice it up!!! It's always a good idea to also pack some of your favorite seasonings to keep on hand when creating your meals.

On-The-Go Shopping List for 14 Days

PROTEIN:

- Boiled eggs (from deli section at local grocery store)
- Morning Star Breakfast Patties (Vegetarian Frozen Food Section)
- Oscar Mayer Deli Fresh chicken strips from Oscar Mayer
- StarKist Tuna Creations (any flavor)
- StarKist Salmon Creations (any flavor)

CARBS:

- Uncle Ben's 90-second Brown Rice (orange bag, rice aisle)
- Steam Fresh Brown Rice (frozen section with veggies)
- Saran-Wrapped Sweet Potatoes for quick microwave baking (produce section near potatoes)

VEGGIES:

- Steam Fresh Veggies (frozen section)
- Pre-cut fresh veggies (Broccoli, Celery)
- Vegetable Crisps (dehydrated vegetables, often found in the nuts section)

Tip: For raw snacking, you can dip in a little hummus, use a little Bolt house Farms Yogurt Dressing (usually found in the produce/salad aisle), or get some all-natural nut-butter to use with the celery. These are borderline foods for the 14-day diet so use very sparingly.

CONVENIENCE MEALS:

Although not the "best", many pre-made foods make your life easy when you can't get your hands on made-from-scratch meals. Choose "quality" over "quantity" and look for lean proteins with veggies that don't have cream sauces or much added flavors.

- o Lean Cuisine Turkey and Green Beans
- o Lean Cuisine Steak Tips with Portabello
- o Lean Cuisine Three Cheese Chicken (acceptable)
- o Kashi Red Curry Chicken (only on 2-carb days)

Stay away from Healthy Choice (all the options don't fit the diet plan, unless you eat around the pastas, rice, or side dishes)

HOW TO: SEMI-HOMEMADE MEALS

Heat up your Steam Fresh Veggies.

If you are on a starchy carb day, heat up your Steam Fresh Brown Rice or Uncle Ben's 90-second Brown Rice.

Heat up your Oscar Mayer Deli Fresh Chicken Strips or serve with 1 packet of StarKist Tuna Creations or Salmon Creations on the side.

Mix together or eat separately for a complete, quick on-the-go meal!

*****For best results, these semi-homemade meals should make up
the bulk of your meals while on the road.*****

CHAPTER 7: HOW TO TRANSITION FROM THE 14-DAY DIET TO LIFE!

Congratulations! You've just completed the 14-day Rapid Fat Loss journey! I hope you're clothes are falling off you, you're feeling better, and are pumped about all the results you've achieved over the last few days.

Now the question begins... How do I keep it going? Well, if you're really loving your results, I suggest doing the 14-day for 1 more week (but no longer than that!). We have a free additional 7 day diet schedule you can grab at bit.ly/14daybook. Because the truth is, the 14-day diet was originally a 21-day plan, but most people got the best results the first 2 weeks, and struggled to do it longer than that. That's why the 14-day diet was born.

But in order to transition back into a more balanced way of eating, there are 5 Rules for Fat Loss that I want to explain first...

THE FIVE RULES OF EATING FOR FAT LOSS

1. You must eat small meals every 3-4 hours (Just like in the 14-day plan).
2. You must build your plate around protein (or healthy fats like nuts, seeds, low-fat string cheese, or greek yogurt for your snacks)
3. You must eat plenty of fruits and vegetables (try to get one with every meal and snack)

a. Fruits are full of vitamins and minerals, fiber and phytonutrients, but they can be high in sugar, too. Try to eat about ½ cup and choose your fruits for your early morning meals or after your workouts, instead of late at night.

4. The best time to eat starchy carbs is after a hard workout and at breakfast. This is the time when your metabolism is the highest, so your body can best use up the carbs, instead of storing them as fat. Carbs will not make you fat, when eaten at the right times and your body prefers carbs as it's main source of energy, so do not cut them out! Just follow the rules.

5. You need to drink plenty of water. We recommend 0.5 oz. per lb. of body weight.

The 14-day Rapid Fat Loss Diet has already given you the framework for eating for life. You've already spent the last 14 days eating small meals that have protein, veggies, and occasionally starchy carbs (when the timing is right). So, continue following the framework of the 14-day diet. I'd recommend following the Plan C (2-carb) days, eating your complex carbs at breakfast and after your workout (see 5 Rules For Fat Loss). You can add your fruits back in but keep it to 1-2 servings per day, and preferably early in the morning.

I know you're probably sick of protein shakes. Therefore, trade your protein shakes for more regular snacks: almonds, string-cheese, baby bella cheeses, celery and peanut butter, veggies and hummus, turkey/cheese/red pepper roll ups, etc. You can still drink protein shakes, but you might want to just do 1 a day.

The 14-day diet is restrictive in order to manipulate fat stores in the best way possible. But now that the 14-day diet is over, it's important to introduce VARIETY back into your meals. Therefore, choose different colors of fruits and vegetables, experiment with recipes that follow the 5 Rules of Fat Loss, and expand your horizons. Variety is the spice of life and a necessary ingredient to keep you on your food plan for life!

Cheers to a sexy, lean body for life!!!!!

The End...???

I see you've made it all the way to the end of my book. I'm so glad you enjoyed it enough to get all the way through! If you liked the book, would you be open to leaving me a 4 or 5 star review? You see, I'm a self published author, and when people like you are able to give me reviews, it helps me out in a big way. You can leave a review for me right here:

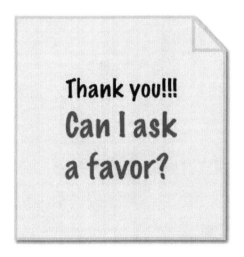

Thank you!!!
Can I ask
a favor?

Thank you for purchasing this eBook.

Connect with Dr. Kristen! Sign up for our newsletter and receive special offers, access to bonus content (including a BONUS 7 days of the 14-day diet plan), additional 14-day Recipes, and info on the latest new releases and other great eBooks from Dr. Kristen Harvey.

Go Here to Sign Up: bit.ly/14daybook

Made in United States
Troutdale, OR
10/11/2023

13626835R00031